Having the Guts to Deal with Bad Shit

My Bowel Cancer Journey

Gemma Farquhar

CONTENTS

Purpose

After my diagnosis of stage 3C bowel cancer that was shortly thereafter restaged to stage 4, it quickly became clear that there was so much information around. It was often hard to sift through; much of it conflicted with each other and there was some (lots) that was not relevant for me—I wanted real people with real stories.

The information was overwhelming and there were some articles that were just frankly scary and did not have much research to back them up. I wanted to understand what the medical jargon was in simplistic terms and I wanted to understand each part of the journey and how it impacted other people whilst understanding each journey is different. It has taken me a long time to get to this point and I still need to remind myself.

The more I spoke about my story the more people leant in to provide me with stories of themselves personally or their loved ones who have been impacted by cancer. When I spoke about it, many people said I was brave but

I have no idea why. It's my story and if it can help other people then it's not brave, it's a necessity.

Had I realised that bowel cancer was not an old person's disease and there was more awareness then I may have got checked earlier, I may have questioned things that were happening—or maybe not; I will never know but I truly believe in telling my story so people can resonate, and to create awareness amongst young people, women especially.

My objective is to use my experience and learnings to create awareness for young bowel cancer sufferers. This is my account which hopefully will assist anyone newly diagnosed or recovering from surgery or chemotherapy and let them know they are not alone.

This has no medical advice or opinions but rather just my experiences from my perspective.

About Me

I have recently been diagnosed with bowel cancer at the age of 35.

I am married with two gorgeous girls who were four and six when I was diagnosed; they are now five and seven.

Growing up, I went to a local school and surrounded myself with friends. I am from Adelaide, South Australia. I am quite organised and have never missed a deadline.

At university I studied Bachelor of Management (Human Resources) and Bachelor of Arts (International Studies) followed by postgraduate studies where I completed my Master of Business Administration. I have worked full time since the age of 19. I have worked in Human Resources for most of the time and started off with entry level roles which continued to progress over time. I felt quite often beyond my years. I like to be constantly busy and have always worked when I was at university and always had a hobby of sorts and been very sociable.

I am often described as strong, brave, willing to give anything a go and assertive. Some people would say I am very loyal, trustworthy, and always willing to be honest and direct in nature—even if the person may not like hearing it. I am not overly affectionate in nature but am very humbled by lovely gestures and the kind human spirit. I have witnessed this so much in the year 2020 where the support has been overwhelming and certainly helped me on my darkest days.

As mentioned, I am originally from Adelaide and moved to Central Queensland at the age of 22 for a job; a year later, I relocated to Sydney which had always been something I wanted to do, given the opportunities Sydney had to offer. I have always been quite ambitious.

I left my last employer in December 2019, after 12 years—it was time to find something new; however, it didn't work out like that, given my diagnosis.

My husband and I met around 12 years ago and have been married for eight years this year. It has gone extremely quickly and we have had some amazing times, including having our children, of course, but also travelling and being surrounded by wonderful friends and family. At home, I am the organiser and completer finisher and my husband has all the ideas; we complement each other in that regard.

We live on the Lower North Shore in Sydney and just love it. Our children, Phoebe and Lily, attend a local school and the community is something that is very much present in the area in which we live. And I can't forget our two dogs, Barney and Betty, who also play a large part in our family.

We are very blessed with everything anyone could possibly need, except I have cancer.

Here is a photo of me in February 2020 overseas and with my family in April 2020 before I was diagnosed. In both photos I had cancer and didn't know it.

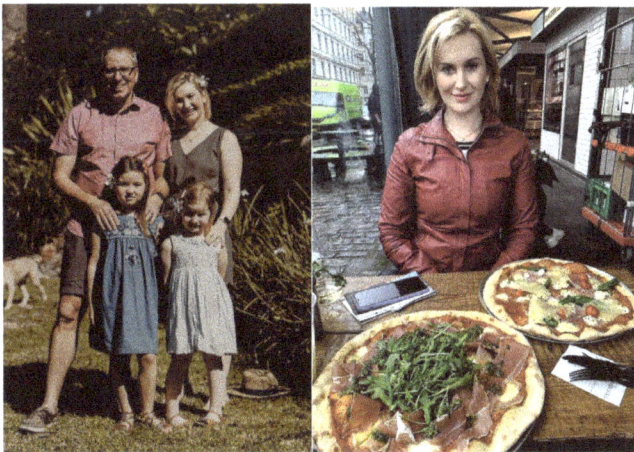

About Bowel Cancer

❧

A ccording to Bowel Cancer Australia, bowel cancer, also known as colorectal cancer, can affect any part of the colon or rectum; it may also be referred to as colon cancer or rectal cancer, depending on where the cancer is located.

The colon and rectum are parts of the large intestine.

The colon is the longest part of the large intestine (the first 1.8 metres). It receives almost completely digested food from the ceacum (a pouch within the abdominal cavity that is considered to be the beginning of the large intestine), absorbs water and nutrients, and passes waste (stool/faeces/poo) to the rectum.

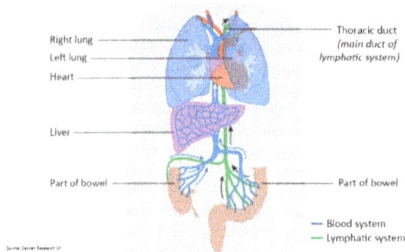

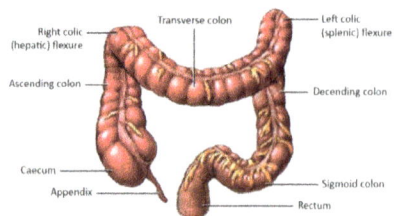

The colon is divided into four parts:

- The **ascending colon** is the start of the colon. It is on the right side of the abdomen. It continues upward to a bend in the colon called the hepatic flexure.

- The **transverse colon** follows the ascending colon and hepatic flexure. It lies across the upper part of the abdomen. It ends with a bend in the colon called the splenic flexure.

- The **descending colon** follows the transverse colon and splenic flexure. It is on the left side of the abdomen.

- The **sigmoid colon** is the last part of the colon and connects to the rectum.

The **proximal colon** is the ascending colon and the transverse colon together. The **distal colon** is the descending colon and the sigmoid colon together.

The rectum is the lower part of the large intestine (the last 15 centimetres) that connects to the sigmoid colon. It receives waste (stool/faeces/poo) from the colon and stores it until it passes out of the body through the anus.

Most bowel cancers start as benign, non-threatening growths—called polyps—on the wall or lining of the bowel.

Polyps are usually harmless; however, adenomatous polyps can become cancerous (malignant) and if left undetected, can develop into a cancerous tumour. The most common type of bowel cancer is called an adenocarcinoma, named after the gland cells in the lining of the bowel where the cancer first develops. Other rarer types include squamous cell cancers (which start in the skin-like cells of the bowel lining), carcinoid tumours, sarcomas and lymphomas.

In advanced cases such as mine, the cancerous tumour can spread (metastasise) beyond the bowel to other organs.

For more information regarding symptoms, prognosis and other important areas I recommend visiting Bowel Cancer Australia https://www.bowelcanceraustralia.org/what-is-bowel-cancer .

My Symptoms

In early January 2020 I had a Friday night pizza with the family. After eating it a few hours later my tummy was rumbling out of control; at 2 a.m. in the morning I needed to empty my bowels and at the same time violently started vomiting—I vomited until every last bit of pizza was out of my body. I instantly felt better after it left my body and resumed to normal the following day. I dismissed this as something being wrong with the pizza.

In February I went away with a friend to Denmark which was amazing; I ate so much and had no issues whatsoever. When I arrived home, in early March, I had some friends over and made some spaghetti marinara which I enjoyed with some bread. Around an hour after I ate it, my tummy was rumbling again and I felt instantly sick, but now two hours after consuming it, I needed to expel it from my body and proceeded to vomit it all up—again, I felt perfectly normal after that but knew it wasn't normal. The following evening, I went out with friends and had dinner but this time instantly knew it needed to come out—it was a rush to get home without expelling it from my body. We were in an Uber and every red light was a nightmare! Again, I felt instantly better after it came out and think I even had a glass of wine after! Bizarre, I know!

The next day or so, I contacted the local doctor and had an appointment. I advised him of my symptoms and he simply said, it's nothing to worry about, it's just a tummy bug. I was not satisfied and asked for a full blood test and some referrals. Had I been working and caught up in day-to-day life, I may not have questioned the advice and may have taken it as correct. Plus, who really likes talking about poo??

As mentioned, given it was a couple of months apart from an episode, I asked for a referral to a gastroenterologist and an allergy specialist. As soon as I had the referral, I made an appointment. Given the joys of 2020 with COVID-19 and the isolation and lockdowns and many people not going out getting check-ups (which hopefully doesn't lead to people not being diagnosed early enough), I was able to get into a specialist with no problem.

The allergy specialist indicated as there was no common ingredient with my food, she did not think I had an allergy. The gastroenterologist indicated I most likely had some digestion issues so put me on some herbal medication for this. I felt better when taking it for a short while. She also sent me for more bloods and requested I do a 'sample', which I did. The sample came back with no additional information. I found out that due to COVID-19, the older technology was used to test the sample as all new technology was put aside for COVID testing.

A few weeks after I did the tests, my tummy was making very loud gurgling sounds and felt a bit crampy at times; I also felt quite bloated. I often describe it to my husband as like a washing machine—I could also feel the food moving in my tummy. I recall sitting on the couch watching TV and the noise from my tummy was so loud. It was moving around, I could feel it. This went on for about two weeks.

At this point, I called the local GP and asked if my results had come back. He simply said yes, they all look fine, a couple of things are elevated but just speak to the gastroenterologist. I then phoned her and advised her of my newer symptoms, which were the inability to go to the toilet at times and slight bloating, but mostly the gurgling sounds—she indicated it could be constipation so put me on some medication for that. Thankfully, she was extremely thorough and was readily available to me. The story continues ...

Finding the Root Cause

◦◦◦

On the 23rd of April, I went for a walk with a girlfriend and had some tummy concerns, more bloating than anything else and a few cramps along with the general feeling of being uncomfortable. I thought the cramps would just disappear like they had on previous days so I continued to persevere as normal. I had only eaten lunch that day which consisted of baked beans on toast as I thought if I was constipated that may help due to the fibre, plus I love them. By nightfall, the cramps had become more intense, my appetite had diminished, and I could not eat dinner. By 6.30 p.m. I started violently throwing up.

We were out on the boat and I was vomiting out of the window, with the first one landing on my husband. I then lay in bed with cramps on the right-hand side of my abdomen and felt extremely hot then cold. I was vomiting every two hours until around 2 a.m. I didn't know what to do and in hindsight, I should have come straight home and gone to Emergency.

First thing in the morning, on the 24th of April, when we arrived home from being away for the night, I had a Movicol, which was previously recommended for constipation, and I called my gastroenterologist as I wanted to tell her what had occurred. I described the pain as 9 out of 10.

On the same day after speaking to my gastroenterologist, she immediately asked me to go for more bloods, have a CT scan and perhaps take some antibiotics if I had some sort of parasite that wasn't previously picked up. It was a weekend so I was so blessed to be able to get into these appointments. Had I lived out of the city or remotely, it would have been far more challenging.

I immediately booked in for a CT scan and did the bloods within the following hour. Amazingly I was able to get a CT scan as they had an opening. In the next hour, the doctor phoned, advising we needed to immediately go into the hospital due to bowel cancer and an obstruction of the bowel/colon (which explained my earlier symptoms). We went into shock and disbelief. I was lying down when she phoned and I was unable to tell Dick. I asked her to advise him of the situation. Dick was outside. I rushed down to him and put him on the phone to the doctor. She advised I had a malignant tumour in the colon and needed emergency surgery as it was blocked. She also indicated she called the surgeon to advise him of my predicament and he was expecting me. I recall every second of this unfolding.

At this point, we told the children I needed to go to hospital for a couple of days to make me better so I would stop vomiting. There was no need to tell them anything else at this point as we were still unclear as to what exactly was happening. It was all very surreal and felt like and still feels like it was happening to someone else.

I immediately packed my hospital bag without any consideration to what I was packing (I have since collated a list of everything needed which can be seen later) and then waited at home for the hospital to call me to get my papers in order for admission and to make sure a bed was available. The wait was excruciating—I coped by letting people know I was headed for the hospital. Dick and I phoned my parents who were also in shock. We committed to keeping them informed every step of the way. After a couple of hours we were on our way to North Shore Private hospital but then changed our journey for the Royal North Shore given the surgery was to be late Friday/early Saturday—and the Saturday was a public holiday. My surgeon called us on the way in and advised us to go straight to Emergency.

Upon arriving at the hospital, we went to the Emergency Room and were seen to after around 30 minutes. I was moved to an open area where there were many people in the process of being admitted. After investigation by several doctors and nurses it was decided that I would have surgery the next morning, Anzac Day, the 25th of April, 2020. I was then moved to a room within the hospital and advised they would come and get me at 8 a.m. in the morning.

Prior to the surgery, I was advised I may need a stoma; I had no idea what this was but didn't care at that point. I later found out that it is where there is an opening in the stomach and poo comes out of it into a bag. It's called an ileostomy or a colostomy, depending if it comes from the small bowel or the large bowel.

Between the evening of the 24th and the 25th of April, I had been taking constipation medication as it was previously thought that could be the reason for my tummy issues. As a result, I was able to decompress my bowel and go to the toilet, a lot! This at the time was unpleasant but it absolutely helped me in the surgery.

Surgery

A fter a restless evening on the 24th of April and the inability to eat or drink anything due to the pending surgery, I woke on the 25th of April with very puffy, red eyes to Dick coming in to where I got wheeled away to the operating theatre. I was in tears and extremely fearful of the unknown. We had been advised that I was going to have open surgery with at least a 10 cm scar and a stoma (I had no idea what a stoma was until this point)—as mentioned above, it's essentially a bag that 'collects' the poo in the event they are unable to resection the bowel again (join two parts back together after the tumour was removed). At this point, I didn't care what was needed—I wanted it OUT.

As I was being rolled into the operating theatre, it was exactly 8 a.m., as promised by the doctors. I met with the Fellow initially who was excellent and she had indicated that there was a possibility that given I had decompressed my bowels, even though it was fully obstructed and a miracle, there may be the option for me to have laparoscopic surgery. The surgery was due to take two hours but four hours later, the surgery finished—I was then in recovery and went back to my room, Ward 8D, Room 28. Dick was there waiting anxiously but had a positive chat with the surgeon who indicated the surgery went well, but at this point we didn't really know what that meant.

It turned out that I did have laparoscopic surgery which meant my healing process was faster as it is far less intrusive. The nurses were amazing in the hospital and my pain management was handled very well. Each day I felt better and better. I had a scar from my belly button up for about 3 – 4 cm and I had four other small incisions from the keyhole components. The scar on my belly button is from where the tumour came out.

On the Wednesday after my surgery, it felt like a waiting game—it was a day where we heard nothing and were in anticipation waiting for my results. The results did not arrive. On the Thursday I did, however, have an action-packed day, including a CT scan in the morning of my upper body—this was to rule out any secondary cancers. The results came back all clear which was a huge positive.

But that wasn't the end—later you will hear about my restaging to stage 4.

Confirmation of Diagnosis

O
ur surgeon then came to get me—by then I had
switched rooms to being with three other people
so she took us to a little room at the side of the ward
and advised us of the details surrounding the tumour. I
had no idea what to expect but given I had been in
Human Resources and she was taking me to a little
room, I didn't think the news would be great. She
advised the following: it was a T4 tumour, with lymph
nodes impacted, plus a lot more that really fell on deaf
ears by that point. I really had no idea what this meant
but understood when she said it was stage 3C.

I felt relief when she said it was stage 3 and not 4 as it
was an indicator it was still contained and not in other
organs. At that point, I felt a sense of relief knowing that
it was in fact treatable and felt at ease for a moment,
until such point of me later googling. To be blunt, I
always had naively associated stage 4 with death. I
didn't realise the gravity of stage 3 or what it meant. In
fact, I didn't realise that stage 3 can be broken down to
a,b,c, depending on lymph node involvement.

The initial types of things I wanted to know were around survival statistics for a T4 tumour (the size of the tumour)what did this mean and what were my treatment options. I started doing lots of reading from sites that I have come to know and love, such as Bowel Cancer Australia and Cancer Council.

We also contacted my friend who has been touched by cancer a few times and is a great source of information and a true inspiration to anyone that talks to her. She is a little pocket rocket!

The next day, Dick and I met with an oncologist that was at the hospital. He advised us of the likely next steps, which included six months of chemotherapy with 12 cycles. Each cycle was to have two hours in the chair and then 46 hours at home with a bottle. I felt confident in the plan at the time; however, it had been two weeks post op and I was yet to see my oncologist so I was feeling like that was the next most important thing after my recovery from the surgery. This was to plan my ongoing treatment—I thought a plan was good and would provide me with direction.

Post Surgery In Hospital

⁓

In the hospital after the surgery, I felt a bit like a pin cushion—my veins are difficult to find so for each blood test and from surgery I had a number of bruises. I mentioned earlier that I was in Ward 8D; initially I had my own room which was divine and reminded me of when I was in the maternity ward after giving birth to my children. Although a vastly different experience. I had never stayed in hospital before having children and had not had other surgery which required me to be in hospital overnight.

Here is a picture of my arms after all the needles I had.

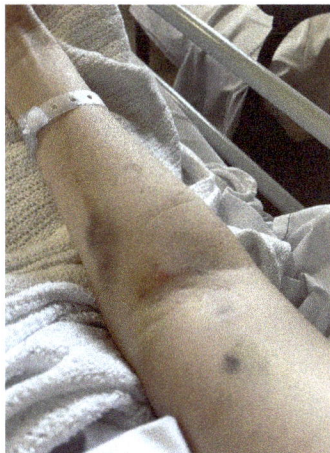

I was in my own room for two nights, then I got transferred to a shared room that held four people. When I went in, it was a bit more confronting as there were three other people in the room. Two were so loud and over the top. One lady to my left was waiting for surgery—she was in the hospital because it was too far for her to go home so she was using it a little like a hotel, a sceptic would say. I heard her life story most nights as she would spend hours on the phone to different people. I suspect she lived by herself and did this in her own lounge; thankfully I had noise-cancelling headsets and an eye mask as she would talk until at least 11 p.m.

Across from me I had another patient—she had completed her surgery and found out she had a benign tumour. She was, however, in pain and the first thing she did when she woke up was demand a nicotine vapor or something to that effect; I could not believe it. She kept making sounds that indicated she was in pain; however, two days later she discharged herself from hospital. I overheard her making a reservation for a hotel and telling people she wanted to get out to have a cigarette and coffee in a comfortable bed ... ! They both left on the same day and it was blissfully quiet with myself and one other older lady who was just delightful and a great support.

Each day in hospital I had bloods taken in the morning and saw my surgeon or his team in the morning to ensure the recovery was going well. Which it was. I had five bandages on and had a drip connected to me which was administering painkillers for the first few days.

I also saw a physiotherapist each day as they assist in determining if you can leave the hospital—they needed me to be able to walk up and down stairs as we have them at home. I did this with no problem by about day five. Also at around that time I would walk around by myself for very short distances and could get into bed and out of bed by myself. Each day there were little milestones that weren't to be taken for granted.

The medical team were very interested regarding when I would do a bowel movement and I did my first one three days post op. I had barely eaten for about six days so it wasn't surprising to not have done one sooner. Post op, I had awful broth followed by apple juice. If I never smell or taste the broth again it will be too soon—it was that bad. I had that then could have soup and any liquid foods. This continued and then I really felt like vegemite toast so that became my new favourite.

In the moments leading up to leaving the hospital, I walked out and felt an overwhelming sense of appreciation and had tears in my eyes. The blue sky, cold wind and a feeling that I was going to be okay rushed over me. I knew now that this had changed me and I was going to have a new appreciation of life.

Telling the Children

❧

On the Saturday following the surgery, I was released from hospital. I was filled with emotion at seeing my two children as they were unable to come to the hospital for the duration of my stay, which was nine days in total, given the COVID-19 restrictions where you are only allowed to have one nominated visitor at a time. This made it challenging in the hospital but thankfully technology was amazing and allowed us to remain connected.

We weren't sure what to tell them and there were so many opinions and literature. As the girls were four and six there were many options, such as not telling them anything, but that was never an option for me. We told them Mummy went to hospital and is better and then told them what I knew—it was that option we went for. My husband was very supportive as we do believe to always tell them the truth, but with truth comes responsibility.

I arrived home just before lunch; the house was decorated with countless flowers and cards which was just lovely. I had pictures drawn for me and the kids were extremely excited which of course filled me with love and affection.

Shortly after arriving home, once the excitement settled down, we casually went in the kids' room and I told them that Mummy went to hospital for her tummy to be fixed, there was a tumour and it's called bowel cancer, but the good news is Mummy feels much better. I also told them that I will need additional medicine and I will do it mostly at home but also some in the hospital—I told them it's called chemotherapy.

Since telling them they have asked lots of questions and I have showed them pictures of things such as the port which I will shortly be fitted with prior to chemotherapy commencing. I often show them my scars or they see them when I am getting dressed and ask questions relating to my stay in the hospital.

I was careful to tell them the words given they will no doubt be used around our household for many years to come, such as cancer, chemotherapy and scans.

As my journey continued, I have moved away from saying 'cancer'—the children didn't realise I was sick which is a good thing; they can see me moving around the house and being 'normal', and that's what I want. I also don't want them in the schoolyard saying 'cancer' as it can have negative connotations and other kids may relate it to death when that's not the case.

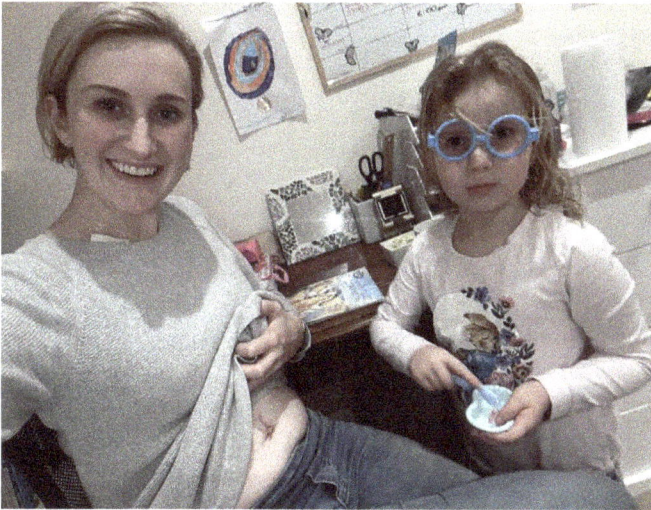

Post Surgery, Pre-Chemo—At Home

❦

It is now two weeks post surgery and I am feeling much better and have more energy than I did before. My support network at home is amazing as my mother and her partner are here for every step. My anxiety is more about the chemotherapy and the unknown about cancer.

We met with my surgeon who was incredibly pleased with how the surgery went and my recovery. He said he will give me the all-clear to proceed with the chemotherapy. He provided me with my pathology results which I had not seen before—there are many words that are unknown to me but there is no sign of other tumours and he collected 30 lymph nodes and eight tested positive. This puts me at the advanced stage of stage 3 (stage 3C) but still lots of positive in sight.

It is now three weeks post surgery and I am scheduled to have a PET scan on Friday. My anxiety over it is quite high given again the unknown and knowing that my last CT scan had bad results.

Today, the 22nd of May, I had my first-ever PET scan. I am still unsure how it differs from a CT; however, someone explained to me yesterday in a support group that I am part of that the CT looks at whole of organs whereas the PET scan picks up any movement of cells. It has been sent to my oncologist and I will get the results on Monday with my plan for the next steps.

I had no idea what to expect in relation to the PET scan. I went into a little waiting room where a cannula was put in; they were unable to get a vein the first time which as indicated is pretty standard. I was then injected with a form of glucose and had to drink three drinks of a liquid that was quite sweet and tasted a little like lemon. I had to lie down for at least 45 minutes whilst the medicine went through my body as apparently the glucose goes to any cancer cells. I then went into the machine. It was quite extraordinary. I didn't even need to take my shoes off and could wear all of my clothes. I went in and said wow, this is exciting—probably the wrong use of words given what they were looking for and the reasons for the scan; however, as the nurse said, perhaps a good first experience was a better way to describe it. Approximately 20 minutes later the scan was done.

Now I have had my PET scan, I am scheduled to meet with the oncologist who will have had an overview of my situation, spoken to my surgeon, reviewed my CT scans, PET scans and full blood work. I have been waiting for this appointment as every question I have results in me needing to ask him and all roads lead to him.

Here is a photo of Dick and I before my PET scan – there is a thing called SCANXIETY – literally Scan Anxiety. It truly does exist and is terrible. The waiting and the wondering.

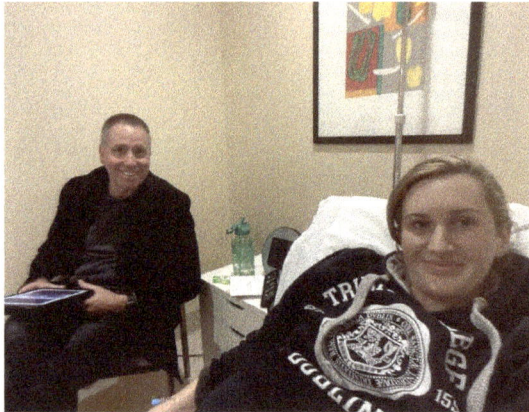

Here are some of my questions; however, I have since had some answered from my surgeon so I won't need to ask him all of them. Many of the questions were from articles I read or some suggestions from various cancer sites and from other people's experiences.

1. How big was the tumour?

2. How many lymph nodes were found and removed?

3. Did you get clear margins?

4. Stage 3—are a, b, c? Scale—where am I at? Does it stay in stage 3 or does it go down/up? Is this defined as early or late?

5. What is the name of my cancer or condition?

6. Is it slow or fast growing? How long would it have been there?

7. Which part or parts of my body are affected? Likelihood it will come up elsewhere?

8. Is it possible to cure or control my cancer?

9. After treatment—likelihood of coming back?

10. When do you know you are cancer free?

11. No family history—but could it be genetic?

12. Will it impact my kids?

13. Genetic testing?

14. Treatment impact my menstrual cycle?

15. Put me in contact with other people impacted?

16. Lynch syndrome?

17. Impact to immune system?

18. Recommended foods?

Treatment

1. What is the aim of each treatment? Is it to cure, control, prevent spread, prevent recurrence or relieve symptoms?

2. What difference will this treatment make to my quality of life, e.g. currently not working but kids?

3. What are the possible side effects of treatment? Can they be prevented or controlled? Are they temporary or permanent?

4. When will I know if the treatment works?

5. What if this treatment does not work?

6. Are there any complementary therapies that I can have?

7. Who are the members of my treatment team?

8. What can I/can't I eat or what supplements can I or can't I have?

9. PET scan?

Clinical Trials

1. Are there any suitable clinical trials available?

2. What would I have to do as part of the clinical trial?

3. What are the possible side effects?

4. What are the benefits and risks for me?

5. Do I have the right to refuse?

6. Can I withdraw from the clinical trial at any time?

7. Are these studies important for me or others?

Four weeks post surgery my critical meeting had arrived. I was so pleased to meet my oncologist and I had heard wonderful things about him. He answered all my questions and I only needed to ask him one or two as he covered everything. I did ask about the PET scan that I was anxious about and he was very confident it showed nothing new and wasn't in any other organs. The sheer relief that took over me is an understatement.

He confirmed what we knew, that I was due to commence chemotherapy. This would be 12 cycles which would happen every two weeks. I would sit in the chair in the Cancer Centre for two to three hours every two weeks and then I would have a portacath put in and have 46 hours at home with a bottle. He then scheduled me to meet with a nurse the following week who advised us of everything we needed to know.

This was the plan before the plan changed. The new plan had me undergoing more intensive chemotherapy and then having major surgery.

Chemotherapy Experience

Five weeks post surgery I met with a nurse at the Cancer Clinic who advised me I would be getting a port fitted the following week with my first round of chemo to follow. It was quite an informative session; however, so much to take in and retain, or at least attempt to. She went over the possible side effects, what to do in case of an emergency, financial information plus all the pharmaceutical needs throughout.

On the 2nd of June, I was scheduled to have my port inserted/fitted/installed—I am still not sure of the terminology so have used a few different ways to describe it. The hospital phoned me on the night of the 1st of June to advise my time for the 2nd. I was to be in hospital by 1 p.m. for a 2 p.m. procedure and would likely be on my way home by around 3.30 p.m. – 4.00 p.m. I went into the hospital at 1 p.m. sharp and signed a form and checked my details. I then got changed into a gown and had a bed in a ward to get onto.

After the first half an hour there, I had sudden stomach pains, was sweating and had clammy hands. I was extremely anxious but had never felt like this before. I sent a text to a couple of friends and put on the TV which was *The Voice*—I did some deep breathing and took control. I then lay down on the bed and waited for the anaesthetist. In the bed next to me the lady returned; she had the exact same procedure as me and I overheard her saying how easy it was—not only that, she looked very well, not with a typical after-surgery look. I was then eager to just 'get it done!' The anaesthetist was lovely and very comforting in relation to putting me at ease. The surgeon then came in and told me what he was doing—essentially putting a port under my skin; he indicated it's been done for many, many years and is a very safe procedure. Shortly thereafter I went into the theatre and had some sedative, or as the anaesthetic said when I asked if it was like a few wines, he said just like a Barossa Shiraz. YUM!

I then felt fine and woke up after about 50 – 60 minutes. I think I may have dozed off, but I can't recall anything. I had a local anaesthetic so I couldn't feel anything where the port was being inserted and when I woke up, there was not that nauseous feeling that I had previously had when waking up from the general anaesthetic—as the local has been wearing off I have had some Panadol which does a great job.

My first night sleeping with the port was challenging, to say the least. I couldn't sleep on my tummy so sat still in slight discomfort. I woke at 4.30 a.m. and one of my dogs was also awake; I then got up and washed my hair in the basin as the surgeon indicated I cannot have a shower for a day or so and I need to keep the port dry. I made a conscious effort to do my hair and make-up—I didn't want to look sick as I am not sick! It made me feel human for the next session, my first chemo session, even though at times it still feels like this ordeal and trauma has happened to someone else. Needless to say, tomorrow I may not make so much of an effort but today, I felt like I wanted to.

The day after my port was installed (today, the 3rd of June), I was scheduled to commence my chemotherapy. Given COVID restrictions, I was unable to have anyone in there with me but Dick dropped me off. He then went to work and Alicia picked me up, which was really lovely. I found the two to three-ish hours went extremely quickly and I watched some Netflix and was trying to take it all in.

When I first walked in, I was greeted by lovely nurses. They were extremely pleasant, welcoming and warm. There were around 25 chairs that reclined; I chose one close to the toilets at the back wall. I had someone opposite me at the beginning and someone next to me for most of the treatment. Upon looking around, there were a few seats taken but it wasn't at capacity. The average age was far older than I am, but I suppose that is to be expected, although cancer does not discriminate and touches people of all ages. I sat next to a lovely lady who is on ongoing chemotherapy and was in good spirits.

Round 1: The nurse explained everything perfectly, like when she was going to touch the port, to when she was putting in a needle, to when the first drug was in, when there was a wash through or when the second one was getting inserted and how long the process would take. She had the bloods that I did pre the port installation as it's a requirement for chemo to have updated bloods each time. I had to go to the toilet a few times too—I told the nurse this and she indicated I had had about 2L of fluid so was happy with that. She was very clear that when I got home, I had to commence washing my mouth out as many times as possible to prevent mouth ulcers which were a common side effect. Each night while I have the 'bottle' on me, I need to also take Movicol plus a steroid each morning, along with any anti-nausea medication. I arrived at the clinic at about 10 and I at 12.30. I was still feeling good at 3.50 p.m. Not feeling cold as yet which is another side effect and am just relaxing and hope I can sleep well and have a walk tomorrow. Upon reflection, I am so pleased that I got the port; it will make this journey far more tolerable as there won't be challenges finding veins each time.

Here is an example of the notes I wrote throughout to go back to my doctor/nurse with:

Day 1: Feel okay, little nausea, at 5.30, slight tingling in feet for five minutes. Water starting to feel cold at 6 p.m., (this meant I couldn't drink any cold water as I would get tingling in my throat which made it unable to tolerate)., woke up at 3 a.m., night sweat woke me, struggled to get back to sleep.

Day 2: Woke tired and face blushed, like warm and a bit red. Slight nausea. Fatigue but not enough to make me sleep. Still mobile and went for a walk. Feeling cold sensation with objects in the fridge (again, this was another side effect, where I had tingling when I touched anything cold)

On Day 3, it was the day to get the 'bottle' removed. I was feeling okay, slightly flushed in the face and I was experiencing minor stomach pains. I asked the nurse about this and she indicated it could be from anything and drugs wearing off. I was still taking anti-nausea tablets just in case I was going to feel unwell.

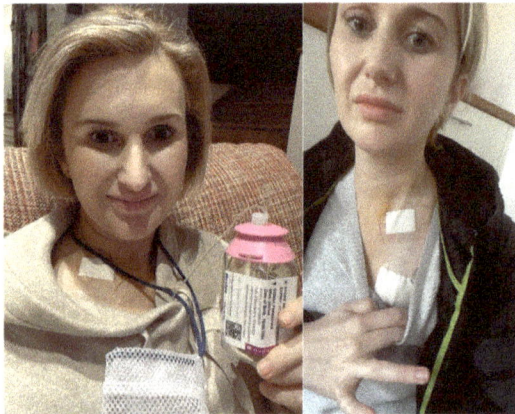

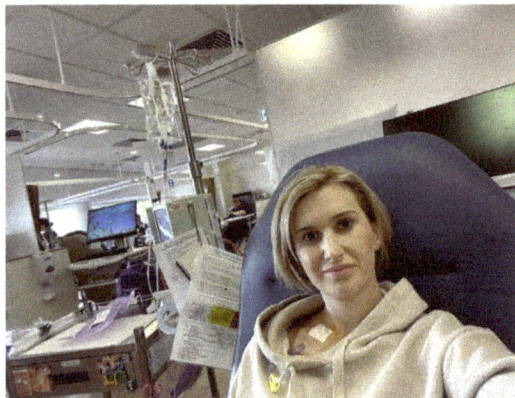

When Things Escalated

How things change. What I am finding out is a plan is never really a plan. I have always known that and adapted but this time more than ever I have needed to understand what is happening and how I am feeling.

On the evening after I finished my first chemo round, the 5th of June, I wasn't feeling great and was taking anti-nausea medication. By the Saturday, I was still feeling unwell, all over. I decided to stay at home all day and rest and was thinking that chemo was just terrible. I have no idea now if it was the chemotherapy; however, by Saturday evening, I started vomiting. It was similar to my initial symptoms when I had the bowel blockage but again, at this time, I had no idea what it was. I vomited about three times, called the emergency oncologist at the local hospital on two occasions and then made the decision to go into hospital.

We arrived at the Emergency Department (ED) at around 6.45 p.m. Upon arrival, given I had chemotherapy, they quickly moved me to a small, isolated room as I was cytotoxic (I had NO idea what this meant but it meant in very simplistic terms that I had chemo drugs still in me) and I had a nurse; he was fabulous! I described my symptoms to him, they inserted a cannula and provided me with a drip. I was having sickness tablets that were helping me to a degree, but it continued to come in waves. I was not feeling well. He also gave me an ECG as I was feeling hot and clammy; this, however, though was more due to the vomiting. I had a lot of bloods taken—more than before and they tested me for more than before. I know now I was tested for my CA and CEA indicators. I am still learning what they are, but they do test for cancer. My results were elevated. I later realised these markers/indicators were going to be very important for my future treatment.

The ED also requested me to do a CT scan. I was unsure why this was required as I had only had a PET scan and CT scan a number of weeks before. A few hours later— by now it was around 1 a.m., I think—the results came back, and I had another bowel obstruction. This time it was likely to be as a result of the scar tissue. I was just shocked. I then had a nasogastric tube put through my nose and I was off all food for a few days to determine if it would pass. It eventually did pass; however, I was in hospital for about five days, five long days.

This to me felt far more isolating than when I was in for 10 days because when I was previously in, I was recovering and consciously getting better each day from surgery. This time, I was waiting around. The doctor who confirmed my bowel obstruction on the night in the ED also mentioned there was a cyst on my left ovary. I was in shock. What did this mean? Shortly thereafter, I was moved to another ward where I stayed for a couple of nights before they moved me to the gastric ward.

Two days after I was waiting on a gynaecological oncologist; however, they never came. My initial surgeon arrived at the end of my bed and told us that he suspected the lump in my ovary was a malignant tumour; he also referenced Krukenberg Tumour and indicated there was a high probability it spread there via the peritoneum. This meant that it metastasised from my bowel cancer.

Again, we were in complete shock and disbelief. Dick and I had no idea what to think, feel or how we could express the emotion. Here we were, knowing previously that I had stage 3C bowel cancer; we knew they got the tumour and had clear margins but I was to have chemotherapy so it would remove anything still there, but with this new information it has literally overnight turned into stage 4 and changed the world as I knew it.

I felt I had been so positive and determined and knew everything would be okay; this new information shocked me beyond anything I have ever experienced. I feel extremely devastated with the news and have cried for the last five days. It is a complete blur. I feel so sad and every time I look at my beautiful baby girls, Phoebe and Lily, I fear that I won't be around for them and their future. This I just can't comprehend. I am determined that I will be around for them and I will do whatever it takes to ensure cancer doesn't win.

After my surgeon told me the news, he also made an appointment to see another doctor, a specialist of this type of spread. Dick and I went to see her on Friday, and she indicated her treatment plan would be to continue with chemotherapy as long as possible and then I would have surgery—this would no doubt mean a hysterectomy, removing the tumour plus anything else seen to the eye and having HIPEC which is a type of chemotherapy. I just digested this and was to have a follow-up meeting with my oncologist the next day as I was shortly due to commence round 2 of chemotherapy. I came home after a tough day to an amazing note from my kids, made out of stones.

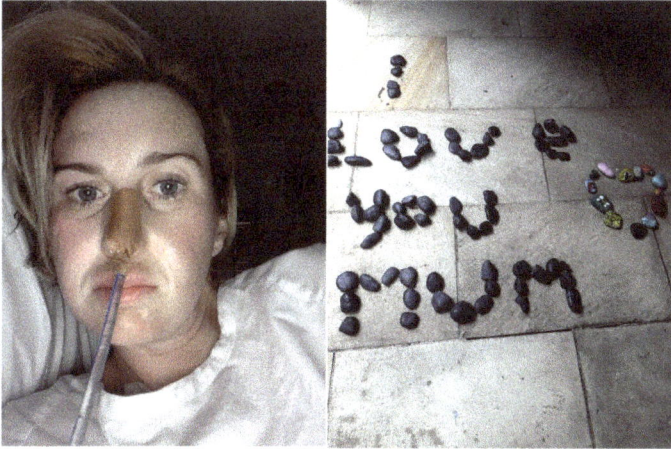

Back To Chemo

Round 2:

I had round 2 of chemo and went feeling very anxious given where I ended up after round 1. I was now on more intensive dugs given the metastatic growth in my ovaries and my pathology results. I met with my oncologist who announced on the day of my round 2 that there are additional side effects from the new chemo which include some nose bleeds and potential hair loss. The new chemo regime was far more toxic (FOLFOXIRI) than the previous one (FOLFOX6); this I think was for two reasons being that I have an aggressive mutation (BRAFv600e) that doesn't always work with treatment and because I had a tumour. This again was a shock but nothing in comparison to the other thoughts I was experiencing. I am starting to learn that each day is different, whether it be emotionally or physically.

Round 3: done!

Round 4: done! Side effects better managed. Pet scan and CT scan completed. Excellent results showing that the treatment is working very well. My hair has started to thin. I get constipation for a few days followed by diarrhoea; these are all side effects. I also get sharp pain at night—again, a side effect, and I can't touch anything cold.

I have finished round 4 of chemo and the days following it are challenging, in that I take a steroid so I can't sleep; I feel like I have morning sickness, hangovers and jetlag all in one. It feels debilitating and I feel like I can't do anything. I have lost weight but feel it's in muscle as I lay in bed for days on end. I then feel 'normal' around five days after the chemotherapy. I have found things to do to occupy my time such as this journal, painting and puzzles.

Round 5: done!

Round 6: done! It's getting harder in some respects and easier in others. I am better emotionally but physically it's a challenge.

It's now after round 6 of my chemo and I have the surgery date of the 17th of September—I am on a break from chemo to prepare my body for surgery. I had previously lost weight with my bowel obstructions and no doubt trauma to the body and stress. My mind wanders constantly, and I am scared of the major surgery. It's called a cytoreductive surgery and HIPEC which I mentioned earlier; the HIPEC part indicates the pouring of 'hot' chemo over me during surgery for around two hours.

I am feeling very anxious and crying a lot. Especially when I think of Phoebe and Lily. I am fearful of the unknown and fearful of knowing I will go into the ICU at the hospital after the surgery. I am also so sad that my children won't be able to come into the hospital because of COVID restrictions, plus I don't want them to see me and remember all the tubes that will no doubt be coming out of me. I have spoken to a fantastic psychologist who has given me strategies to deal with the anxiety and to compartmentalise it.

It's now nearing the end of July and I can say I have turned a corner mentally. It took me about six weeks to grieve the information and stop thinking about dying. It has been so, so tough. I have had days where I didn't want to speak to anyone, others where I would just cry and feel sad, depressed and think about dying and of course my babies and wanting to be around for them.

The cancer has certainly changed my life and my thinking; it has made me more present with my children and husband and appreciate every single second I have with the people I love. I have an amazing psychologist who has helped me put in place strategies to assist in my thinking. The strategies that have helped me are to write down my thought or to recognise it's a thought— this helps in separating myself from the thought.

The other strategy that has helped was to name all my thoughts and pretend it's a book title; mine was *Journey to Death*—all my thoughts were about dying, my funeral, and planning for my babies and husband. The psychologist indicated it's a boring book, it's been read, and all the people are the same, the chapters are the same and to put it back on the shelf. Visually it has helped.

I now feel like I have a plan to fight this cancer away and although it is long and challenging, there is hope and determination. I again feel positive like I did when I received my first diagnosis. This does come and go in waves though.

I don't like my children seeing me in bed, lying down constantly, and at times that makes me feel sad but as soon as I think that I know they are extremely resilient, and they know Mummy has medicine. Regardless, the chemotherapy is helping fight the cancer so it's all worth it.

A few weeks ago, I was almost hooked on googling again to understand more about my diagnosis—I have realised it's a fine line between knowing and not being an expert vs not knowing anything and relying on the experts. I have decided now I am not going to google anymore as it is quite frankly scary; the statistics for my type of cancer seem extremely daunting. I have a specific mutation/DNA to the tumour—this I googled which again scared me like never before. A few people have been helpful in reassuring me that it's better to know exactly what you are dealing with to treat it accordingly.

Second Surgery—Peritonectomy

Today it's the end of August and I have my specialist appointment with the surgeon on Monday. I can't wait for it. I am extremely fearful and scared of both the surgery and having cancer whereby people die from it. I can only think of being here for my girls. Today, I clicked on a news article that had someone who passed away; it was reported he was stage 3 and progressed to stage 4 and had a four-year battle. This has rocked me; I now need to focus on the positives and turn off to articles like this, it's just too sad and confronting.

I can't wait to meet with my surgeon as I have been very anxious with the build-up and just want to know what they are planning to do. Everything I know has been via the internet or other people's stories so I can't wait to hear it directly from the surgeon. I am tired, I am anxious, and I have been crying a lot, given the unknown. I keep thinking of Phoebe and Lily and again, just need to be around for them and watch them grow old. It was Phoebe's birthday this week; it was a lovely day, but I couldn't help but think, what if I wasn't here for the rest of them? It's those thoughts I am trying to deal with. I have a very good psychologist who helps me get through those thoughts with a number of strategies. Everyone is different and her style has certainly worked for me. I have written notes for my kids so every day I am away at the hospital, they can read a note from me. This was particularly hard to write, I wanted it to be special and memorable plus I wanted them to get excited. I couldn't help but thinking though, what if I didn't come back after the surgery.

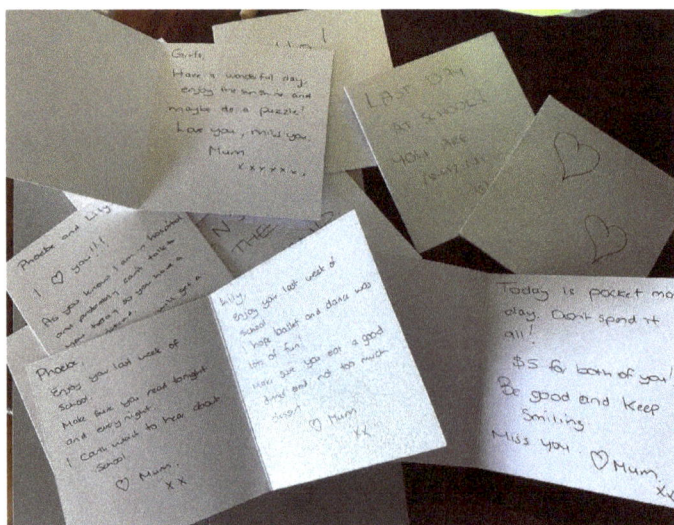

I am required to have this surgery as I understand cancer can travel a number of ways, and via the peritoneum is one way, given the new tumour is on my ovary—there is evidence which suggests it spread via the peritoneum, hence this surgery. The surgery itself hasn't been around for decades; in fact, it has only become the norm since around 2013 and has only been happening at my hospital for three years. There is a full unit at the hospital, and I have felt supported in the lead-up to meet my surgeon; I have had a dietician contact me along with a psychiatrist and a social worker.

I met with my surgeon a couple of weeks ago now and I have needed that time to digest everything she told me. Essentially, she told me I was having a full hysterectomy, removing my appendix, peritoneal and omentum, plus potentially removing my gall bladder and spleen. She indicated that there was a 30% chance of major complications and 20% chance of requiring a colostomy bag. I would be without a belly button and when I wake from surgery, she said I will have a number of tubes in my nose, mouth, drains from my stomach and a catheter. I went into a spin. I was not ready for all this information. I began crying in the appointment; Dick was with me and we were both shocked. I needed time to digest this information. I knew I was facing major surgery but the extent of this was huge; perhaps I had not realised it as I was previously undergoing the chemo so was just concentrating on that. I have come to realise surgeons and doctors are very direct in their style and nature and tell it all as worst-case scenarios. Not sure if this is reality or my reality at times, given where my head is at sometimes.

A week after meeting with the surgeon, I had pre-admission which consisted of me meeting people for four hours. I needed an ECG, X-ray and blood tests, plus I met with a clinical nurse to take me through the day ahead, the anaesthetic doctor to discuss what type of anaesthetics would be administered throughout the operation, the surgical doctor who relayed what the process was, the nursing case manager and a stoma therapist. The last one, being the stoma therapist, was the most confronting. The nurse drew a 'dot' on my skin in the event I needed one—it would guide the surgeons where to put it. I am praying I don't need one as already the journey and recovery will be tough and I would be lying if I didn't say I want my body back to the new normal, even though it will be without a belly button.

I also met with the oncologist who advised me regarding the HIPEC part of the operation; this is where they pour 'hot' chemotherapy over me for an hour at the end of the surgery. I had previously thought it was longer, but they confirmed the time. One of the bad things about google is you sometimes get conflicting information.

The day prior to surgery quickly approached after what felt like a long wait. The day before surgery I was instructed to have clear liquids only and then in the afternoon have PICOPREP which is a drink to clear your bowels—needless to say, after the consumption of the drink, within an hour I was ready to sit on the toilet and clear my bowels! Aside from the prep drink, I also needed a drink each hour which was to carb load my body, to provide me with energy throughout the surgery. I am not exactly sure what it does but I did as instructed. I didn't know how I was feeling: I was anxious, I was nervous, I was scared of the unknown and fearful of the surgery. I wanted to be on the other side, feeling grateful.

The night before the surgery, surprisingly I slept well although it was a late night, and then the next morning my alarm was set for about 4.30 so I could have another special drink, this one to carb load to ensure my body had enough energy for the duration of the surgery.

Day of surgery: We woke up, my bag was already packed and we were ready to go—I was very emotional and just wanted to cry. It was extremely hard saying goodbye to the girls and to Mum. It's one of those things that I wish I didn't need to go through, I wish no one had to go through it, but in saying that, there were no other options. I needed this surgery and this surgery would be my best case for long-term survival. We arrived at the hospital after finding a car park nice and close; this point may not seem like much but being the wife of Dick, it means a lot and keeps the peace, parking is said to be very important!

We walked into the hospital, got checked for the COVID test and then proceeded to where we needed to check in. They asked for my Medicare card and within 10 minutes of waiting a nurse called Dick and I to another room to ask a series of questions, both personal and medical related. He was helpful but I was in no state to chat; after about another 10 minutes after all the questions, I was then taken to change rooms where I was required to get into a hospital gown and then proceed to a waiting area for surgery.

Given the length of peritonectomies, I was the only operation happening that day. It was excruciating saying bye to Dick as I had no idea when I would wake up or what I would wake up to. I was rolled into theatre by about 8 after talking to the anaesthetists and nurses.

They then put me out, put tubes in me (a NG tube) and drains, plus a central line which I was to learn would later be the source of nutrition being pumped into my body. All these things happened when I was asleep.

At about 5.30 p.m. I was woken up, I can't recall where I was or who I spoke to upon waking, I did ask the time and was provided with that though I didn't know if it was a.m. or p.m. Prior to the surgery I was told that they may keep me asleep for the evening and wake me in the morning depending what time the surgery finished. I cannot recall if I was woken up in a waiting room or if I was woken up in ICU; either way, my first recollection thereafter is being in ICU.

Time in ICU—post peritonectomy: It was a different world—one I had never seen before. The noise, the culture, the illnesses, and the dynamic and energetic nurses that were by my side the whole time. The nurse I had on my first night was excellent. I felt extremely attended to and felt she was very competent; she would clean all my wounds, check my blood pressure, make me comfortable, warm and ensure that I was progressing as needed.

When I was in ICU, I can't recall what day, but my surgeon came past—I was very excited to see her. She said the surgery was a success and she was very happy with it. It turns out that all the cancer was in the one place, in my pelvic region, so the outcome of the surgery was a peritonectomy, omentectomy, resection of the bowel from where it was previously cut—apparently this is where things are likely to return so they take a safety approach—removal of my appendix and I had a full hysterectomy.

The ICU was tough and I would be lying if I said it was easy. I couldn't walk for four days—I would get dizzy when I tried to walk and felt nauseous, I felt fatigued, I was in and out of pain although it was managed very well. I couldn't move and was turned around and washed. I couldn't sleep, the constant beeping was awful. The tubes, the machines and the medicines—I really had no idea what was going on but trusted in the medical employees who were excellent. I had drains in my stomach that were attached to me along with stitches from under my breasts to my vagina. I was in ICU for a total of five nights, so I left on the following Tuesday that followed the operation on the prior Thursday. I felt overwhelmed with leaving as the nurses had solely been responsible for me and I wasn't sure I was ready to be more independent.

Aside from not feeling ready to leave ICU as I had only just been able to get out of bed for about three steps and this was aided by the physiotherapists holding me up. I felt completely and utterly reliant on other people, for the first time in my life. I had a catheter for me to wee in, I had a tube that was feeding me my nutrition, I had drains coming out of my stomach and I had a significant incision right down my insides.

My last night in ICU was one to remember: I recall this guy who was more interested in his social environment and next party or where he was getting his next coffee from—am sure he is a competent nurse but he lacked emotional intelligence. I am grateful though that all the other nurses demonstrated such care for what they did.

Now I was ready to go to the ward, the next chapter began.

Ward—following ICU: Following ICU I was taken to the colorectal ward where there are patients with colorectal (bowel) issues. I went to my own room initially but that didn't last long, the next day I moved to a shared room. I was okay with that but was equally exhausted. I had previously not had much sleep in the ICU so needed to catch up on it badly. My mind at this point was going through a mix of emotions and feelings as I felt helpless, that I couldn't do anything; I could barely move and I was 36 years old. How could I let myself be like this? Those feelings did not last for too long; I quickly moved on and thought of Phoebe and Lily and how much I was missing them but realised they were having a lovely time.

I am writing this now on day 10 in the hospital and I feel a bit unsure of what to type, largely because the last few days have been a blur. Each day I have felt there have been little baby steps in the right direction.

In the ward you quickly get into a routine of bloods, drugs, food, sleep and repeat. After a couple of days in the ward, I was put on a clear fluid diet and then it gradually increased when my body could handle it. I hadn't eaten for over seven days and had intravenous nutrition given to me. As the intravenous nutrition was turned down, the food intake started to increase. The drip ended up coming out. I still, however, had two drains in my stomach along with the central line.

After a couple of days my catheter came out; I then got a urinary tract infection—yuk! This was, however, being treated with antibiotics and was on the mend.

A couple of days after that, my bloods came back a bit low so I received a blood transfusion. This was a bit bizarre as I never thought I would need one but grateful for the people who donate blood on a regular basis. It truly is lifesaving for people.

On a daily basis, I had the physio come and visit me; this was a blessing in disguise because without it I probably wouldn't have had the motivation to move. The physio each day pushed me further and further to walk or to move my legs and regain some strength. It is incredible how quickly you can lose your fitness and strength from major surgery. It made me feel weak and unsure if I would ever regain what I lost and be 'normal' again.

As the days went on the surgeon indicated I would go home by the end of the week; this initially freaked me out as I didn't feel ready but it soon turned into excitement as I realised that I could do more and that the hospital wasn't the best place for me.

I was becoming increasingly sad at the prospect of this cancer never going away, meaning I would not be there for my two babies when they grow up—and this thought continued to consume me. Coupled with the fact that of the people in my ward, one was terminal (although she was in her mid-80s) and two others had the cancer return for a second time—this is another one of my fears so it just wasn't becoming healthy for me to be there.

I needed to leave.

Here are some pictures of my scar post 4 months of surgery along with the cords attached to me in ICU and drains that were connected to my stomach for days post-surgery.

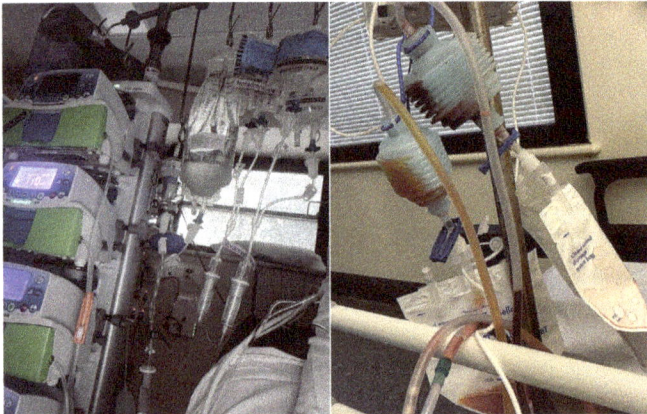

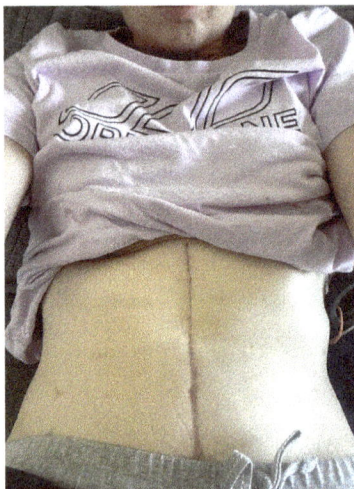

Coming Home

The day came when I was discharged. Dick picked me up from the hospital in the morning and my paperwork was quickly finalised. I was quite anxious but excited about returning home. I wasn't sure how I would be, given my mobility, or lack of, but knew it was the best place for me to recover as I wasn't getting much sleep in the hospital. Once Dick picked me up we walked about 500 metres down the road to where the car was parked; this was intense. I wasn't able to walk without stopping. I needed constant rests to muster up the energy.

Coming home was a lovely feeling although my girls were still on school holidays and away with friends and their grandma—the house was very quiet but it enabled me to get some of my confidence back.

After a couple of days I was missing the children like crazy and they soon came home. I was overwhelmed with joy to see them as my greatest fear is not being here for them as they reach all of their milestones in life.

I am now five weeks post-surgery and am feeling okay. I pushed myself too much the other day with my movement so am in a bit more discomfort than I have been which impacts my mobility. I am now very slow.

I was surprised that my hair continued to fall out after my surgery so I bought a wig but ended up not using it as it just felt too uncomfortable and I didn't feel like me. It was a fun process though – the kids loved it as well as you can see by the picture of Lily wearing the wig. I ended up just cutting my hair very short.

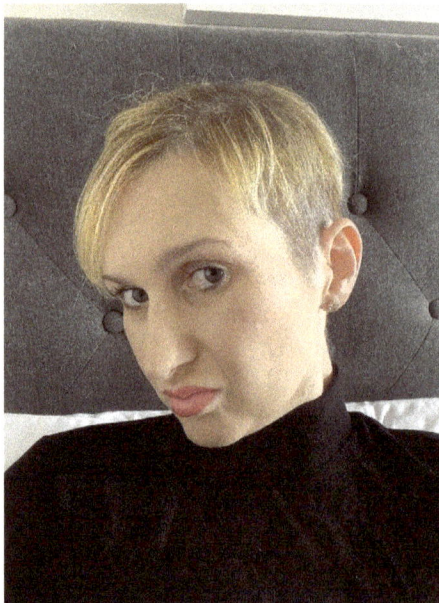

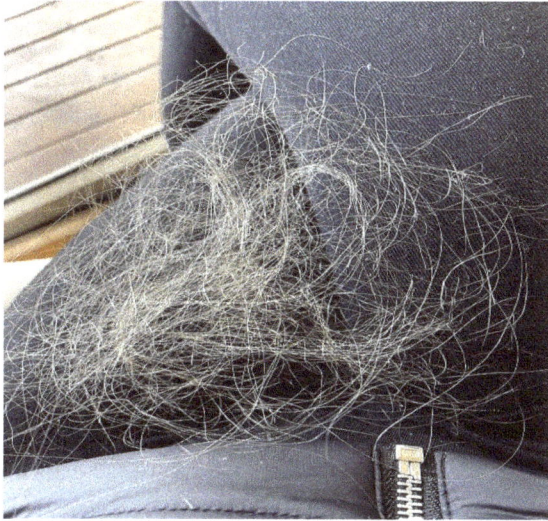

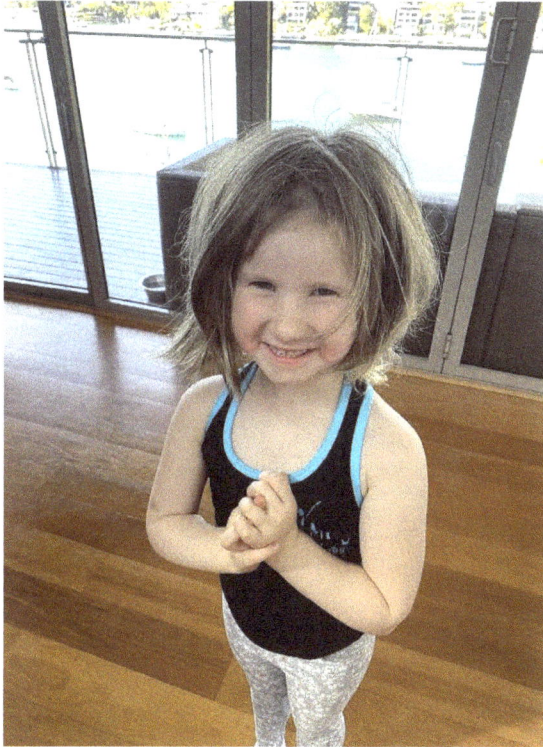

Histopathology Results

❧

After a week being home, I was following up my pathology results; subsequently, I received the results via email and was awaiting a call from the surgeon to provide an overview of what it all meant. It was a four-page document but the summary is below. When I read the operation report it stated that there was a left side tumour on my ovary, a little one on my right ovary along with some more spots at the initial location where I had my first tumour on the bowel. I was shocked that there was more as I wasn't sure how this could happen.

Upon receiving my pathology results, it indicated there was just the tumour in my left ovary and the majority of the cancer cells were dead. This was good news but interpreting it is challenging. My surgeon said it was positive but obviously still couldn't reassure me regarding my future which I find tough, but I understand it completely.

I have had the time now to look at my pathology from my first surgery and my pathology from my second surgery—they raise a number of questions for me which I have sent to my oncologist who I am meeting with on Friday, which is five weeks post-surgery. I should have an indication of what comes next for me in regard to scans, bloods and chemo.

Surgery 2 – Pathology Summary

SUMMARY

1– 14. Hysterectomy, bilateral salpingo-oophorectomy and peritonectomy specimens as above:

- Metastatic mucinous adenocarcinoma,
- In left ovary, predominantly acellular mucin pools and necrosis with scant amount of viable tumour cells
- Adhesions elsewhere in the multiple peritonectomy specimens
- Consistent with good response to therapy (TRG1)

I don't understand lots of it but sought information from my oncologist; after all, it's their job to interpret the results. I felt like I needed clarity as this is regarding me; I do appreciate I have an amazing oncologist so I am sure he will answer my questions and put me at ease. I am also going to get a blood test prior to my meeting with him on Friday; this will allow me to get an indication of my tumour markers which will hopefully put me at ease and acknowledge that they got all the cancer. I am not sure I can cope with any more surprises in this regard; mentally it is a challenge.

I had my meeting with my oncologist; it was very positive. He indicated my pathology was favourable as there was less cancer than they initially thought via the operation and no lymph nodes were impacted. He answered all my questions and was very thorough. I am due to start chemotherapy again in the next week which will see me doing six more rounds. I am going to go on the 'less' toxic one so there should be fewer side effects.

My oncologist indicated this is adjuvant 'mop up' chemo and they are going for a cure. I was thankful I was operable and that I had a good response to the chemotherapy. This was good news although can never be guaranteed. I also got a result to my tumour markers CEA and CA19.9. My CEA was down to 0.8 and my CA19.9 was 5. At its peak my CEA was up to 42 and my CA19.9 was 158 so you can see how much they have reduced as a result of the chemotherapy and surgery. I couldn't believe this news. It was like a normal person. I felt extremely blessed and in shock—it was surreal; this was six months to the day of diagnosis.

I was cancer free.

After meeting with my oncologist, I had a post-op appointment with my surgeon. She felt my tummy to see how it was healing and we had a general conversation. She was quite positive and said I would be monitored closely and can find a new job when my chemo has finished. This was amazing to hear—I was going to be okay.

Although my brain continues to have 'what if' scenarios but I am learning to cope with them.

Back To Chemo—Mop Up

On the 3rd of November I commenced my chemo again; this was the less toxic (if that's a thing) version. As I walked into the clinic, I got weighed which was standard and then I chose a chair that was free. The nurses are lovely and were once again very welcoming. I got connected to my first drug and then an overwhelming emotion came back to me, it took me back to the beginning of this journey. It felt like I was/am still sick and didn't feel different to the last times, but it should have felt different, or so I thought. I am hoping and praying that this is some sort of insurance policy to kill off anything that may be left but again hopeful nothing is left. I have been googling a lot and need to stop it; it's like a fixation—I want to know as much as possible, but it doesn't help me. I was meant to be cancer free, but this made me feel terrible. Like I was still sick. I couldn't understand the feelings.

As I write this, today I am still connected to my bottle. I am not feeling as unwell as I did previously. I wrote this and then my anxiety got worse; I was so down. I thought

I would feel better but instead I wanted to question everything. I don't know if it was the steroids or the fact that my body has been through so much. The neuropathy has also impacted me this round. Something I need to discuss with my oncologist.

Another round nearly down and round 8 in a fortnight.

This week, I had round 8. My fingers and toes are starting to feel tingly most of the time which is a bit strange. My oncologist reduced the dose of the chemo this round by 25% which meant that I have also had less side effects. When I got into the chair on Monday, it was awful. I was so down and so anxious—I couldn't help but cry the whole time. I saw my oncologist who was and still is excellent; no one could rationalise this situation. I am scared. I am scared that I won't be here for my babies and get a huge sense of being overwhelmed by this. My googling this round has been particularly bad; I just want to find something good about that mutation I have. I can't find anything. I need to think of the positives: I have had a great response to chemo and I have had surgery. My oncologist tells me I need luck; hopefully my bad luck has been and gone.

I have been struggling.

Round 9 in a fortnight. I hope to make the most of my week of feeling 'normal'. Round 9 went okay except I had bad neuropathy; it's hard to type!

Round 10 and 11 have happened with no oxaliplatin. This is the drug that causes neuropathy. This has made it particularly easy compared to every other chemo infusion.

Round 12 today. I went in today with Dick, although with the COVID restrictions he could only come to my appointment with my oncologist. Prior to this appointment I had a CT scan; it's my first one post-surgery. I was hopeful it would be all clear.

It is clear where the previous cancer was but there are some nodules on my lungs that need monitoring; I am hoping it's inflammation. They need to rule out that it's not cancer so I am having another scan within a month.

This has again shattered me but I am thankful that they are very thorough. Leaving the chemo place was bizarre, thinking and hoping and praying it's my last chemo but not really knowing.

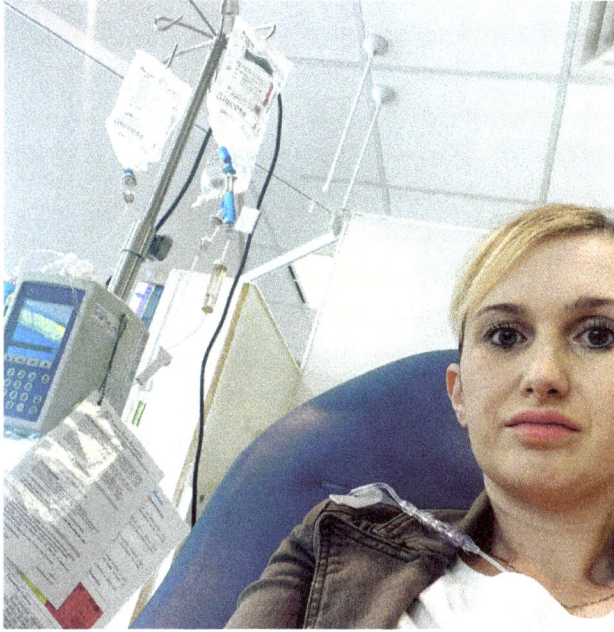

Other Information

CLINICAL TRIALS

When I was first diagnosed or misdiagnosed with stage 3, my oncologist spoke about an aspirin trial. Without knowing much, it was basically to see if taking aspirin would reduce the likelihood of the cancer returning. I did not do much investigation with regards to this before I was diagnosed with stage 4 when the tumour was found in my ovary.

That being said, I am going to undertake the MOST program which is conducted by the Garvan Institute which looks at rare cancers and the DNA make-up of them. They are an amazing research facility. I am excited to be part of this program as it will provide other opportunities for treatment if needed. I was required to have a phone screen, complete paperwork and do bloods. The people at the centre will also get my tumour and test it. It takes about eight weeks to get any results. Around eight or nine weeks later, today, the 14th of September, I received my results; we didn't learn anything new about the tumour so that's a good thing as far as we already knew it and I was being treated for it. My oncologist indicated there were other mutations but they were common with cancer and wouldn't change the treatment.

MY EDUCATION JOURNEY

After hearing I had cancer, I really had no idea what it meant—yes, I had heard of cancer and a number of my friends had cancer and were fighting fit and others weren't as fortunate. I did a bit of googling but it didn't provide me with a clear and simple explanation so I ended up watching a kids' YouTube video that simply said, they are bad cells in your body that multiply quicker than the good ones. This helped me when I explained it further and got more and more information that was less easy to simplify. This was the foundation of all the other components to come.

I learnt so much along the journey and would learn to understand and question. I would mix up my education by talking to other people and hearing their stories with a bit of googling but ultimately I would save all my questions for my doctors. Reality is, I want to know I am going to be okay but regardless of how much education

I receive, I am not going to get an answer. It will be what it will be.

I would rely also on sites such as Bowel Cancer Australia who had all the information I needed.

COMPLEMENTARY THERAPIES

Today I had my first acupuncture since being diagnosed. I loved it! It made me feel relaxed and helped me with my nausea. There are so many different therapies and I encourage anyone to do their own research and find out what works for the individual.

Along the way I have also seen a naturopath and dietician.

Four weeks after my first surgery and I went back to do exercise with my trainer. Reality is, I could have done it myself but I enjoy the social interaction and the support. It was very light weights and a little walk. After four weeks with what my body endured, the amount of muscle and as a result strength and fitness that I lost was very surprising—it was a lot. I am now absolutely motivated to get both my fitness and my strength back before I commence chemotherapy.

What has motivated me the most is exercise and the acupuncture and I look forward to getting into recommendations from my naturopath. Another thing that has helped me along the way was looking at positive quotes or affirmations. I have attached some of these (at the back) so you can read them and hopefully they will help you too! I am not sure of the source of them all, however they are readily available and more often than not, I found them on Instagram.

SUPPORT GROUPS AND INFORMATION

When I was still in hospital, one of the things I thought was important to me was to be connected to others who have had a similar experience, but I wasn't sure how to go about it. I initially started googling support groups and came across two in particular: the Bowel Cancer Australia site where there is peer-to-peer support and the SAN Cancer Centre which is part of a hospital in the Northern Beaches in Sydney. I initially joined the SAN Support Group—this was an online Zoom call; because of COVID-19 it was not able to be face to face. This suited me. The first call was the Thursday following me being discharged from hospital and it was the first time I said out loud that I had cancer. It was quite confronting. I found the two hours on the call very insightful—there were many other sufferers on the call at various stages regarding the disease and life stages.

I was about 30 – 40 years junior to the others on the call so I was mindful of using their wisdom of experience to provide me with as much information as possible. Some of the lessons I learnt was to keep a diary of how I am feeling to report back to the doctors and to ensure I get a copy of every single blood test and scan to become aware with what the doctors see. I now have a dedicated Excel spreadsheet in chronological order of each meeting, specialist appointment and links to the required documentation. This made me visualise the illness as more of a project that I could tick things off on as I go along.

I also contacted Bowel Cancer Australia in regard to their peer-to-peer support and they put me in contact with a girl of 25 who was diagnosed with bowel cancer the year prior. She is doing well and had genetic issues; however, it is her story to tell. I found it helped me speaking to someone again who was or had been through similar events. Similarly, I know someone who is now based overseas who was diagnosed five months prior; however, at stage 4. I am finding it very helpful sharing my journey with her and asking those silly questions but knowing that everyone has the same silly questions, hence the importance with writing down my recollections.

Upon my restaging to stage 4, Bowel Cancer Australia also put me in contact with other people who have had the same surgery I am having. One of them is doing amazingly well and an inspiration—her cancer is completely gone and she is living her best life. The other one I have only spoken to on one occasion and her cancer came back; I wasn't quite ready for that conversation at the time but equally I want to be there for her.

Cancer Council of Australia is also a source of information and I also reached out to a counsellor to try everything and anything that is available to determine what may or may not work for me.

The counsellor was quite good—at first I was sceptical; however, she asked me a number of questions around how I was feeling but more pointed, like did I blame myself. I was taken aback by this but upon talking to other people it is quite common to say, why me? I, however, have not felt that way; instead, I am more focused on the here and now and recognise it's just one of those things! Reality is, I do have it so what do I need to do to make it go away? I will continue this as I progress through the chemotherapy as I am sure not all days will be perfect.

Throughout my journey I would often become obsessive with finding out information. This would include me googling any articles I could and putting in different search words that may or may not result in a more favourable article. I would also be on Facebook sites that would have people posting a number of questions— sometimes these helped me and other times they just made me feel worse. It became increasingly clear that everyone's journey is very different but it took me a long time to actually realise that. Even with someone who would describe the same type of cancer as me, including the mutations and location, it was still different. I am now finally at ease with this and although I remain on some of the Facebook sites and still google, I feel like it's more of a science research project as opposed to the what's happening to me and looking for answers that google won't give me. It won't predict my future; I just need to have faith.

I find I get fixated on a topic and search it at length; this has included 'survival statistics' and prognosis but what is also evident is that prognosis for one I have, i.e. BRAF mutation, is poor but then the pathology indicated all cancer was gone so this could potentially be better prognosis. It's so confusing so I have just learnt to read it, but read it understanding that these articles may or may not be relevant to me, and again it's my own journey.

People would often recommend books to me to read. I skimmed a couple but I found it more depressing reading about cancer when I had cancer—all the recommendations, what was right and what was wrong, what you should do, how you should feel, what you should eat, how much exercise you should do and an ongoing list of natural remedies. It was all consuming and I found it better to put them down and perhaps it was better for people close to me to read as opposed to me, but it's very personal and up to you to decide what you want to do.

CREATING AWARENESS

Bowel Cancer Australia also has on their website stories of people who have been impacted; most cancer sites do so I was inclined to write a short story regarding how my symptoms were diagnosed. I then received a call to see if I would be interested in being a little bit of a spokesperson for the month of June, as June is Bowel Cancer Awareness month. Of course, I said yes as it is so, so, so important to me that people understand what I went through, how it wasn't diagnosed as early as it could have been and how I hope that others can get to it sooner.

In hindsight, my bowel movements most likely had changed to be inconsistent—not in time but more so texture. I have since learned it should always be 'sausage' like. However, given I had two children, a full-time job—it became my new normal and was just part of the way I was (or so I thought).

TIPS ALONG THE WAY

- Always ask questions.
- Keep a record of all documentation.
- Look at it like a project plan.
- Always accept or ask for help from family and friends.
- Ask for blood tests to always be sent to you.

- Have water before bloods.

- Keep a diary of any symptoms you may experience.

- Try and take it a day at a time.

- Do as much or as little as you like.

- Exercise as much as you can.

- Be positive! (easier said than done, sometimes you just need to cry and that's okay too)

EMLA: I learnt about this early on; it is cream to put on the area where the chemo needle is going to go in—it is a numbing cream so takes away any pain. This was a good one to get!

Look Good Feel Good: This is an amazing NFP charity. They provide cancer patients with a number of workshops for hair and make-up with the premise of look good, feel good! It was nice getting my package in the mail full of make-up suppliers. I am yet to book into a session but appreciate what they do and their contribution. My hair is falling out still at the moment so at some point in the near future I will need to look for tips re a wig.

What is needed in hospital:

- Pyjamas

- Face wash

- Toiletries

- Hair brush

- Make-up if needed

- Slippers and socks and undies

- An outfit to leave hospital in

- Phone chargers with a long cord

- Books/crosswords or anything to pass the time

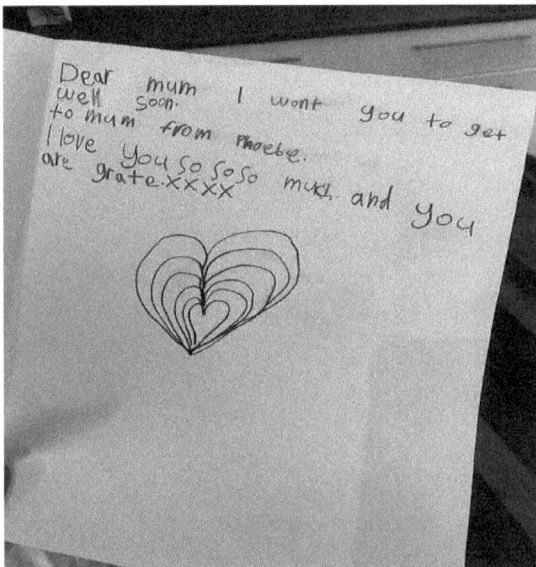

Family And Friends And Thank You!

❧

Having close family and friends around for me is very important. It's important for a number of reasons, such as being able to talk through what is happening, how it happens and to be positive and optimistic (as hard as it is at times).

When I was in hospital a number of friends dropped things off at the hospital as they were unable to come in due to COVID-19. This consisted of things such as magazines or flowers, not to mention things for me to take home to the kids to keep them occupied. By the time I came home a number of friends had dropped off food, I had a florist worth of flowers, plus a number of gifts. These were all lovely and the cards were very heartfelt and made me realise that it is important to surround yourself with people that truly care.

I have had friends who have offered to walk with me up and down the street whilst I have been recovering from surgery and others who have sent lovely text messages and phone calls. I have reached out to other people in the same situation which has also assisted me to cope.

As time goes on, it's quite interesting: it almost becomes the norm for people—some you hear from constantly and others not at all or very sporadically. It truly is a long-haul journey.

I have days where my mind wanders and around 100% of the time, it's about my two baby girls. I just want to be there for them both for the next 70 years.

As I lay in the hospital ward after my second surgery (the peritonectomy) I woke to a lovely message from Katie; it was very short and sweet and again reiterates how much everyone's support and ongoing support is needed and appreciated.

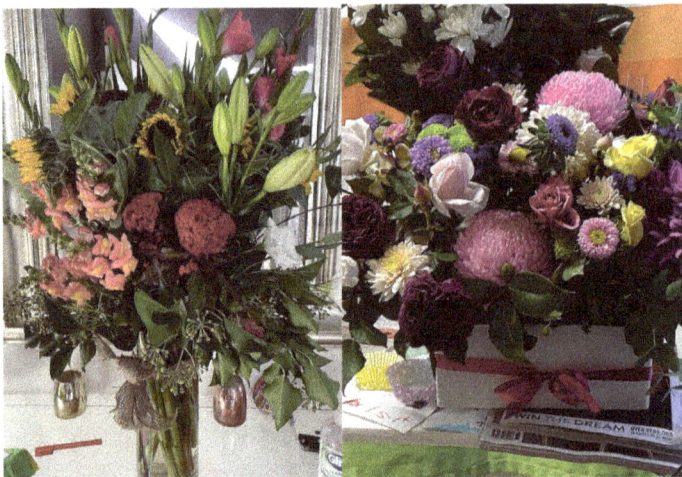

Where To From Here?

I have finished my chemotherapy and had a recent scan; there are some nodules in my lungs but we are monitoring them at the moment. This will be my new norm as I am to get scans every three months and will be kept under close surveillance. I am scared but I have chosen to put my energy into finding my new normal and spending quality time with those around me.

The next two years will be tough as I hope and pray that the cancer stays away, this is the critical time for monitoring as there is a likelihood that if it returns, it will return within two years.

I hope to return to work and create further awareness as it is so incredibly important that people talk about their stories, talk about any symptoms. I had no idea this disease could happen to young people but it absolutely can. I hope my story helps people going through the same or similar journey or helps family members of those impacted.

In the past 10 months I have had over 80 medical appointments and four hospital visits. It has been gruelling. It has been the only thing on my mind.

My advice to all is to persist and if something feels wrong, please investigate. It often goes unnoticed in younger people until it has advanced in stage, when it is not as easily or as successfully treated.

I am going to finish by writing a note to Cancer which I wrote after my surgery but while I was undergoing my last chemo sessions.

Thanks for reading.

Letter To My Cancer

Cancer, you are the overwhelming word that I struggle with.

I had always been scared of you, scared of getting you, and I have always associated you with older people and people who die. I know quite a few people who have been touched by you! Then there I was, less than a year ago, getting the diagnosis that I have cancer.

Bowel cancer, to be exact.

Bowel cancer that also went into my ovary.

Cancer, you have tried and tested me. My mental and physical strength. The ongoing feeling of nausea throughout the chemotherapy.

My obsession with googling and Facebooking— trying to find positive articles of people who have the similar aggressive mutation of a BRAFv600e.

It has taken me time to realise that you, Cancer, are different for everyone and there is no one person the same. Cancer, you have led me to hospital on four occasions and two major surgeries.

The pain has been significant.

Cancer, you have made me fear not being here for my children and husband. That pain is the hardest. You have made me question my values, my reason for living, and made me extremely grateful for any milestones, birthdays and special events.

I am so much more present than I was before you. You are bad but you have also taught me to have faith. You have introduced me to many great people, including other patients and frontline medical practitioners.

At times, you made me feel like I was a number, not a person, but I have learnt to take control, control where I own my journey through questioning the doctors and making sure I am across every blood test and result. I have now finished my final six chemo sessions and I want to say goodbye to you, Cancer, goodbye to you for good. I will not miss you but I will forever remember each and every step of my journey. I want to pass my learnings on to other people so they too can deal with you and then farewell you.

YOU, CANCER, CAN FUCK OFF!

*This picture and story was used in June to promote Bowel Cancer Awareness month, the other photos pictured were from an article that was again published for awareness in some local newspapers.

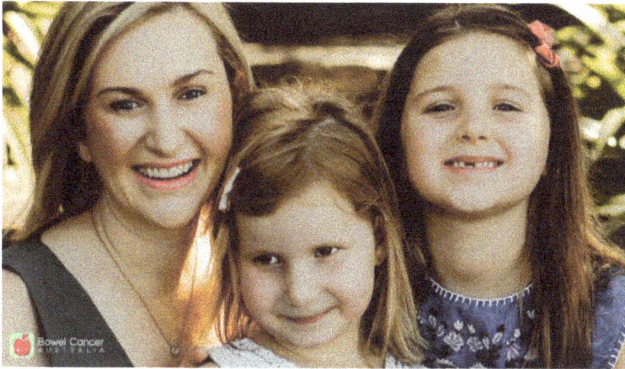

Bowel Cancer Australia
537 followers
1d · Edited · ⊕

Symptoms remain NOT NORMAL despite the NEW NORMAL.
Ahead of Bowel Cancer Awareness Month (June), we are urging Australians that despite uncertainties due to COVID-19, early detection of the disease cannot and should not stop, even during a pandemic.

Gemma, diagnosed with Stage 3 bowel cancer, said: "At 35 with two young children aged 4 and 6 - bowel cancer was the last thing on the doctor's mind but I knew something wasn't right when I began vomiting after food. The doctor simply put it down to a 'tummy bug'."

"I had my surgery when COVID-19 was in full swing, but the hospital was amazing with everything quarantined and isolated. The only impact COVID-19 had on me in hospital was the inability to see my children for 9 days given only one nominated visitor at a time was allowed."

"My message to everyone - please present if you have symptoms as they can't be ignored, and the best chance of survival is getting it early. Additionally, please persist with doctors and ask the questions or seek referrals to specialists if you feel something is wrong."

Read Gemma's story here: https://bit.ly/2AX8FiP

Click link to read more about our 'Not Normal' story: https://bit.ly/3eo4riN

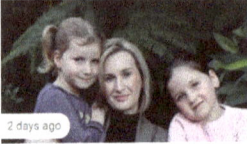

Wait times for bowel cancer checks ...
heraldsun.com.au

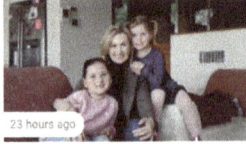

Bowel cancer wait just became more ...
noosanews.com.au

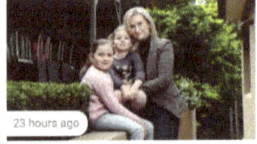

Bowel cancer wait just became more ...
noosanews.com.au

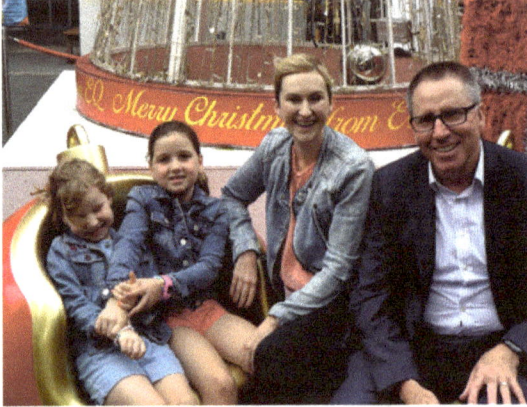

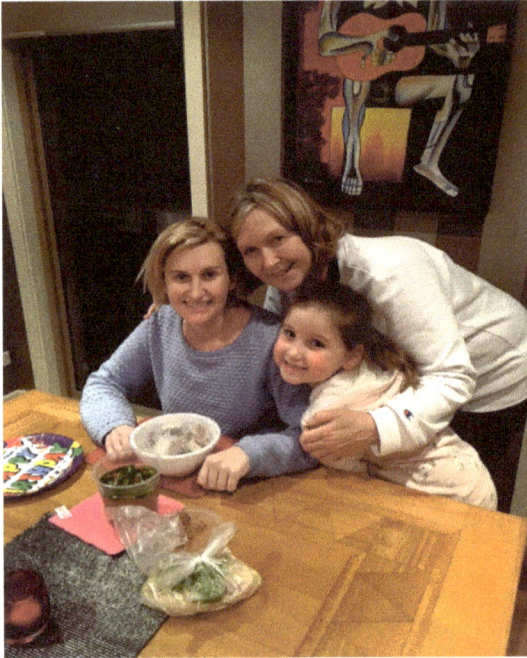

Breathe, darling.
This is just a chapter. It's
not your whole story.

S.G. Louie

ONE DAY
YOU WILL TELL
YOUR STORY
OF HOW YOU
OVERCAME WHAT
YOU WENT
THROUGH AND
IT WILL BE
SOMEONE
ELSE'S
SURVIVAL
GUIDE

One day at a time is all
we should be dealing with. We
can't go back to yesterday and
we can't control tomorrow,
so live for today.

If you can stay
positive in a negative
situation, you win.

You're a fighter. Look
at everything you've
overcome. Don't give
up now.

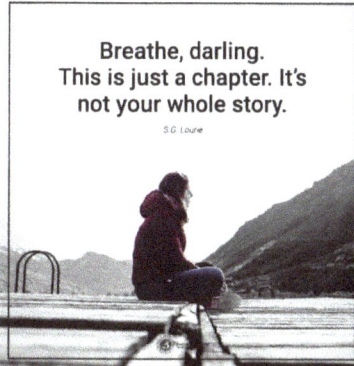

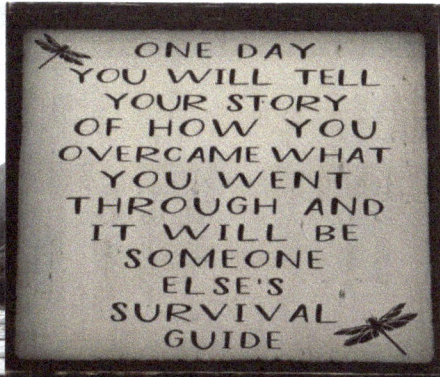

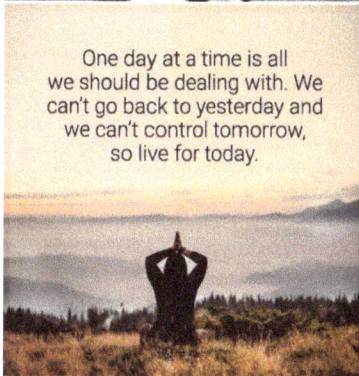

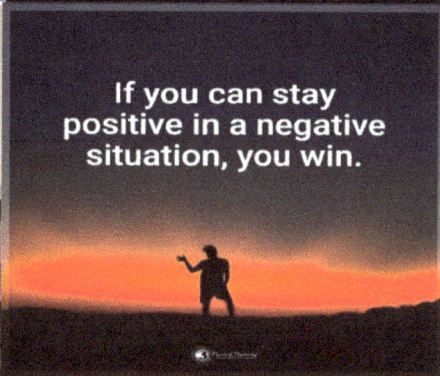

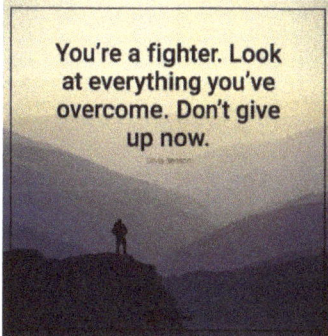

Stop being afraid of what could go
wrong and start being positive about
what could go right.

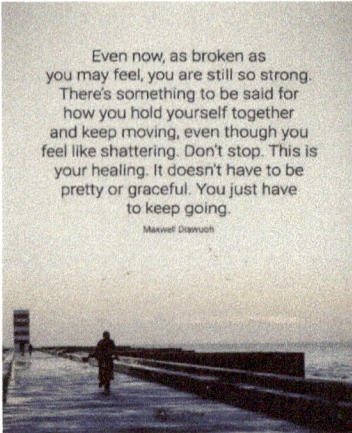

Even now, as broken as you may feel, you are still so strong. There's something to be said for how you hold yourself together and keep moving, even though you feel like shattering. Don't stop. This is your healing. It doesn't have to be pretty or graceful. You just have to keep going.

Maxwell Diawuoh

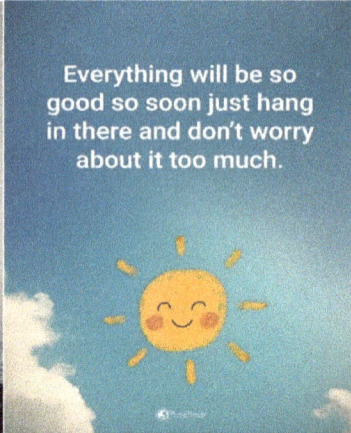

Everything will be so good so soon just hang in there and don't worry about it too much.

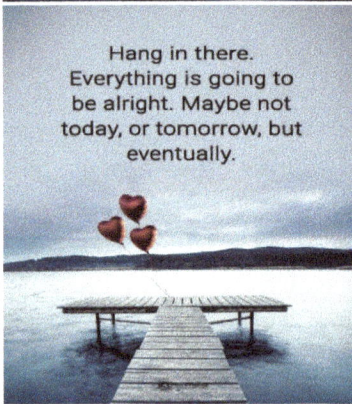

Hang in there. Everything is going to be alright. Maybe not today, or tomorrow, but eventually.

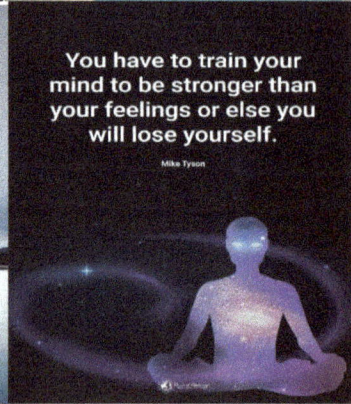

You have to train your mind to be stronger than your feelings or else you will lose yourself.

Mike Tyson

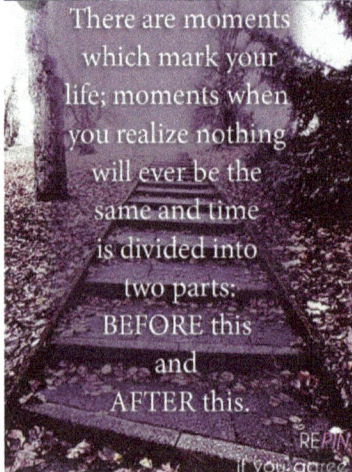

There are moments which mark your life; moments when you realize nothing will ever be the same and time is divided into two parts: BEFORE this and AFTER this.

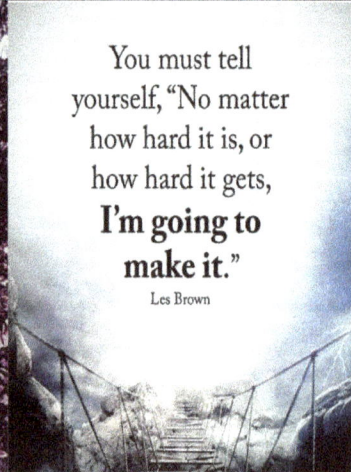

You must tell yourself, "No matter how hard it is, or how hard it gets, **I'm going to make it.**"

Les Brown

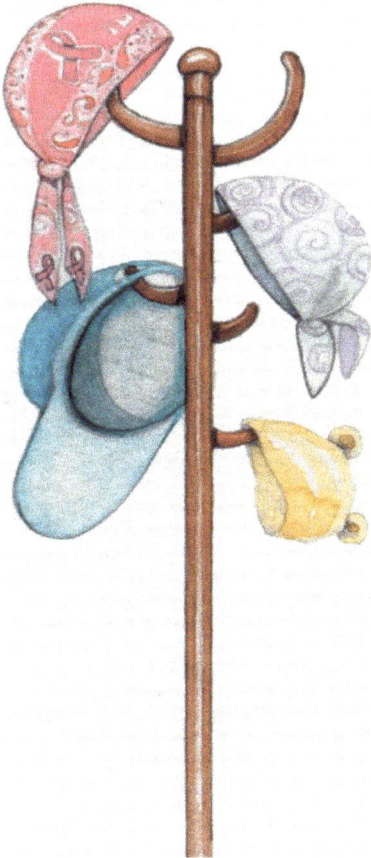

chemo

It's a big tough cure
for a big bad disease.
It's caring so much
about life and those
you love that you're
willing to put yourself
through the wringer.
It's remembering that,
with every passing
minute, every day that
goes by, you're that
much closer to being
done ... with cancer.

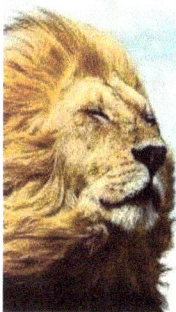

Courage
doesn't always roar.
Sometimes courage is
the little voice at the
end of the day that
says I'll try again
tomorrow

Mary Anne Radmacher

You don't always
need a plan. Sometimes
you just need to
breathe, trust, let go, and
see what happens.

Mandy Hale

Overthinking ruins
friendships and relationships.
Overthinking creates
problems you never had.
Don't overthink, just overflow
with good vibes.

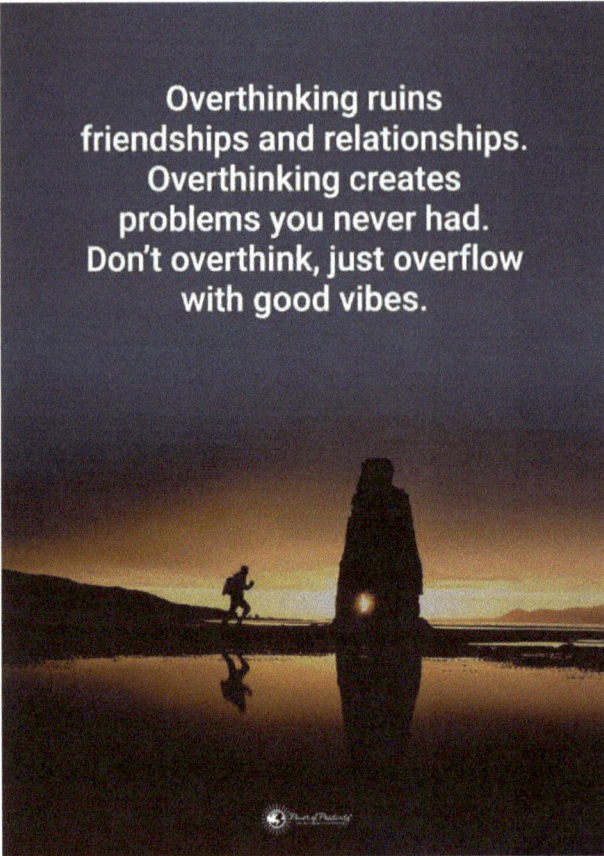

NIKOLAI LENIN

"You are braver
than you believe,
stronger than
you seem,
smarter than you
think, and twice
as beautiful as
you'd ever
imagined."

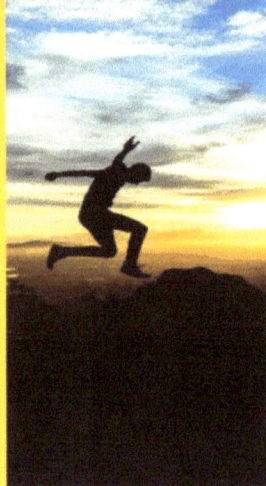

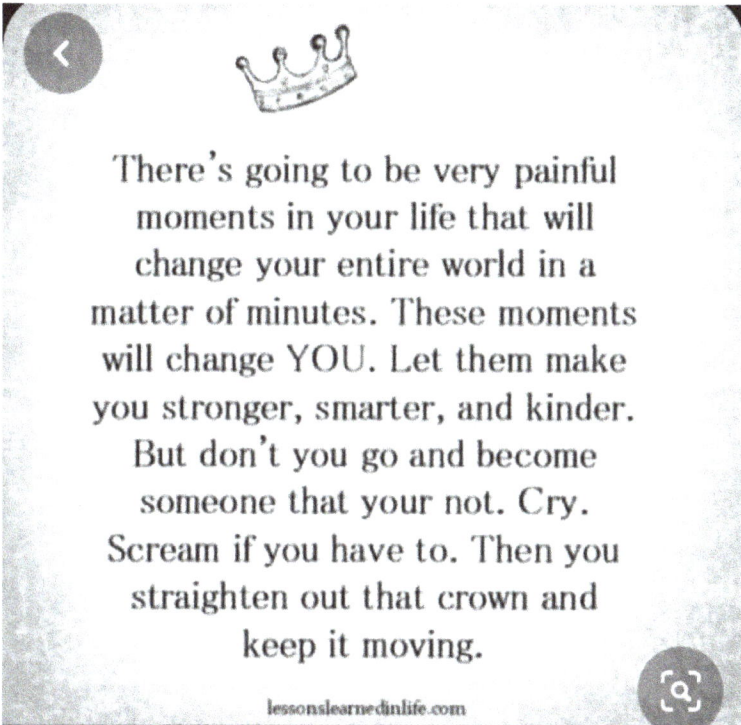

There's going to be very painful moments in your life that will change your entire world in a matter of minutes. These moments will change YOU. Let them make you stronger, smarter, and kinder. But don't you go and become someone that your not. Cry. Scream if you have to. Then you straighten out that crown and keep it moving.

lessonslearnedinlife.com

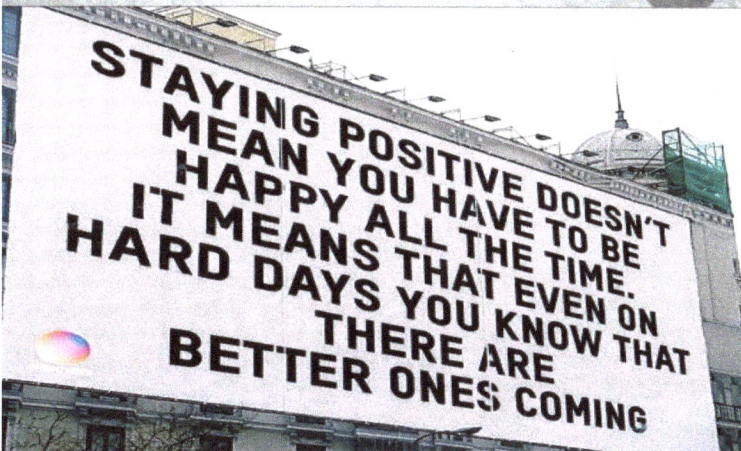

STAYING POSITIVE DOESN'T MEAN YOU HAVE TO BE HAPPY ALL THE TIME. IT MEANS THAT EVEN ON HARD DAYS YOU KNOW THAT THERE ARE BETTER ONES COMING

www.ingramcontent.com/pod-product-compliance
Lightning Source LLC
Chambersburg PA
CBHW041300040426
42334CB00028BA/3106